T0281101

Cambridge Elements ≡

Elements of Improving Quality and Safety in Healthcare
edited by
Mary Dixon-Woods,* Katrina Brown,* Sonja Marjanovic,†
Tom Ling,† Ellen Perry,* Graham Martin,* Gemma Petley,* and
Claire Dipple*
*THIS Institute (The Healthcare Improvement Studies Institute)
†RAND Europe

STATISTICAL PROCESS CONTROL

Mohammed Amin Mohammed
Faculty of Health Studies, University of Bradford

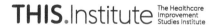

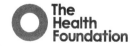

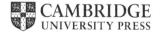

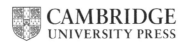

Shaftesbury Road, Cambridge CB2 8EA, United Kingdom

One Liberty Plaza, 20th Floor, New York, NY 10006, USA

477 Williamstown Road, Port Melbourne, VIC 3207, Australia

314–321, 3rd Floor, Plot 3, Splendor Forum, Jasola District Centre, New Delhi – 110025, India

103 Penang Road, #05–06/07, Visioncrest Commercial, Singapore 238467

Cambridge University Press is part of Cambridge University Press & Assessment, a department of the University of Cambridge.

We share the University's mission to contribute to society through the pursuit of education, learning and research at the highest international levels of excellence.

www.cambridge.org
Information on this title: www.cambridge.org/9781009521291

DOI: 10.1017/9781009326834

First published 2024

A catalogue record for this publication is available from the British Library.

ISBN 978-1-009-52129-1 Hardback
ISBN 978-1-009-32680-3 Paperback
ISSN 2754-2912 (online)
ISSN 2754-2904 (print)

Statistical Process Control

Elements of Improving Quality and Safety in Healthcare

DOI: 10.1017/9781009326834
First published online: February 2024

Mohammed Amin Mohammed
Faculty of Health Studies, University of Bradford

Author for correspondence: Mohammed Amin Mohammed,
profmaminm@gmail.com

Abstract: Statistical process control methodology was developed by Walter Shewhart in the 1920s as part of his work on quality control in industry. Shewhart observed that quality is about hitting target specifications with minimum variation. While every process is subject to variation, that variation can arise from a 'common cause', inherent in the process, or a 'special cause' which operates from outside of that process. This distinction is crucial because the remedial actions are fundamentally different. Reducing common cause variation requires action to change the process; special cause variation can only be addressed if the external cause is identified. Statistical process control methodology seeks to distinguish between the two causes of variation to guide improvement efforts. Using case studies, this Element shows that statistical process control methodology is widely used in healthcare because it offers an intuitive, practical, and robust approach to supporting efforts to monitor and improve healthcare. This title is also available as Open Access on Cambridge Core.

Keywords: statistical process control, control charts, run charts, funnel plots, monitoring healthcare

ISBNs: 9781009521291 (HB), 9781009326803 (PB), 9781009326834 (OC)
ISSNs: 2754-2912 (online), 2754-2904 (print)

Contents

1 Introduction

This Element begins with an intuitive illustration of the two types of variation that underlie statistical process control methodology: 'common cause' variation, inherent in the process, and 'special cause' variation, which operates outside of that process. It then briefly describes the history, theory, and rationale of statistical process control methodology, before examining its use to monitor and improve the quality of healthcare through a series of case studies. The Element concludes by considering critiques of the methodology in healthcare and reflecting on its future role.

The statistical details for constructing the scores of charts found in statistical process control methodology are beyond the scope of this Element, but technical guides are signposted in Further Reading (see Section 6) and listed in the References section.

1.1 Understanding Variation by Handwriting the Letter 'a'

In this section, we use the process of handwriting to demonstrate the ideas that underpin statistical process control methodology. Imagine writing the letter or signature 'a' by hand using pen and paper. Figure 1a shows seven 'a's written by the author. While the seven letters appear unremarkable, what is perhaps remarkable is that even though they were produced under the same conditions (same hand, date, time, place, pen, paper, temperature, light, blood pressure, heart rate, and so on) by the same process, they are not identical – rather, they show controlled variation. In other words, even a stable process produces variation or 'noise'.

In seeking to understand this controlled variation, it might be tempting to separate the 'a's into better and worse and try to learn from the best and eliminate the worst. This would be a fundamental mistake, since the conditions that produced them were the same, and so no 'a' is better or worse than its peers. The total variation seen in the seven 'a's has a common cause, which is inherent in the underlying process. Efforts to improve the quality of the letters need to focus on changing that process, not on trying to learn from the differences between the letters.

What changes could we make to the underlying process to reduce the variation and improve the quality of the 'a's? We could change the pen, paper, or surface, or we could use a computer instead. Of these suggestions, we might guess that using a computer will result in marked improvements to our 'a's. Why? We can draw useful insight from the theory of constraints, which compares processes to a chain with multiple links.[1] The strength of a chain is governed or constrained by its weakest link. Strengthen the weakest link and the chain improves. Strengthening other links simply uses up resources with no

(a)   (b)

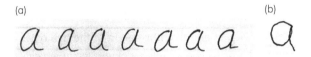

Figure 1 Handwritten letter 'a'

benefit. In the handwriting process, the weakest link (constraint) is the use of the hand to write the letter. The pen, paper, light, and so on are non-constraints; if we change one of them, we will not make a material difference to the quality of our 'a's. Switching to a computer to produce our 'a's, however, will see a marked improvement in performance because we would have overcome the weakest link or process constraint (handwriting). So, a stable process produces results characterised by controlled variation that has a common cause, which can only be reduced by successfully changing a major portion of the underlying process.

Now consider the 'a' in Figure 1b. It is obviously different from the others. A casual look suggests that there must be a special cause. In this case, the author produced the letter using his non-dominant (left) hand. When we see special cause variation, we need to find the underlying special cause and then decide how to act. Special cause variation requires detective work, and, if the special cause is having an adverse impact on our process, we must work towards eliminating it from the process. But if the special cause is having a favourable impact on our process, we can work towards learning from it and making it part of our process (see the Elements on positive deviance[2] and the Institute for Healthcare Improvement approach[3]).

In summary, the handwritten 'a's demonstrate two types of variation – common cause and special cause – and the action required to address each type of cause is fundamentally different. The origins of this profound under-standing of variation are described in the next section.

1.2 A Brief History of Statistical Process Control Methodology

This understanding of variation – which underpins statistical process control methodology – comes from the physicist and engineer Walter Shewhart.[4] His pioneering work in the 1920s at Bell Laboratories in Murray Hill, New Jersey, successfully brought together the disciplines of statistics, engineering, and eco-nomics and led to him becoming known as the 'father of modern quality control'.[5]

Shewhart noted that the quality of a product is characterised by the extent to which the product meets the target specification, but with minimum variation. A key insight was his identification of two causes of variation:

- *common cause variation*, which is the 'noise' intrinsic to the underlying process
- *special cause variation*, which 'signals' an external cause.

This distinction is crucial: reduction of common cause variation needs action to change the process, whereas special cause variation needs identification of the external cause before it can be addressed.

Shewhart developed a theory of variation which classified variation according to the action required to address it, turning his abstract concept into something that can be measured in the form of statistical process control methodology. The methodology has proven to be very useful in efforts to improve the quality of manufactured products. Its migration to healthcare appears to have happened initially via applications to quality control in laboratory medicine in the 1950s.[6] Since the 1980s, the use of these methods has continued to expand, especially in monitoring individual patients,[7] for example following kidney transplantation,[8] for asthmatic patients,[9] and for patients with high blood pressure.[10] Statistical process control is now used across a wide range of areas in healthcare, including the monitoring and improvement of performance in hospitals and primary care, monitoring surgical outcomes, public health surveillance, and the learning curve of trainees undertaking medical or surgical procedures.[11–14]

2 What Is Statistical Process Control Methodology?

Statistical process control methodology offers a philosophy and framework for learning from variation in data for analytical purposes where the aim is to act on the underlying causes of variation to maintain or improve the future performance of a process. It is used in two main ways:

- to monitor the behaviour or performance of an existing process (e.g. complications following surgery), or
- to support efforts to improve an existing process (e.g. redesigning the pathway for patients with fractured hips).

By adopting this methodology, the user is going through the hypothesis-generation and testing cycle of the scientific method, as illustrated by the plan-do-study-act (PDSA) cycle (see the Element on the Institute for Healthcare Improvement approach[3]), supported by statistical thinking to distinguish between common and special cause variation.

Box 1 highlights various descriptions and features of common versus special cause variation. In practice, a graphical device – known as a statistical process control chart – is used to distinguish between common and special cause variation.

Box 1 Features of common versus special cause variation

Common Cause Variation	Special Cause Variation
• Is caused by a stable process (like writing a signature) • Is sometimes referred to as random variation, chance variation, or noise • Depicts the behaviour of a stable process and affects all those who are part of the process • Can only be reduced (but not eliminated) by changing the underlying process • Can be predicted, within limits, with the aid of a statistical process control chart • The variation between individual data points from a stable process has no assignable cause extrinsic to the underlying process	• Is variation which is extrinsic to a stable process arising from an assignable cause • Can be favourable or unfavourable • Does not affect all those who are part of the process • Is a distinct signal which differs from the usual noise of the process • Is sometimes referred to as non-random variation or a signal of systematic variation • Signals of special cause variation can be seen on a control chart but need further detective work to identify the assignable cause

In the next section, we look at the three main types of statistical process control charts commonly used in healthcare.

2.1 The Statistical Process Control Chart

Statistical process control methodology typically involves the production of a statistical process control chart (also known as a process behaviour chart) that depicts the behaviour of a process over time and acts as a decision aid to determine the extent to which the process is showing common or special cause variation. Scores of control charts exist,[15] but three main types have been used successfully in healthcare:

- run charts[16]
- Shewhart control charts[17]
- cumulative sum (CUSUM) charts.[18]

This section introduces the three main types of charts by using systolic blood pressure data from a patient with high blood pressure (taken over 26 consecutive days at home before starting any corrective medication). Figure 2 shows the blood pressure data over time using a run chart, a Shewhart control chart, and a CUSUM chart.

- The run chart (top panel) shows the behaviour of the blood pressure data over time around a central horizontal line.
- The Shewhart chart (middle panel) shows the same data around a central line along with upper and lower control limits.
- The CUSUM chart (bottom panel) doesn't show the raw data, but instead shows the differences between the raw blood pressure data and a selected target, accumulated over time.

As Figure 2 demonstrates, several charts can usually be used to examine the variation in a given data set. In general, run charts are the simplest to construct and CUSUM charts are the more complex. This highlights an important point: although several (appropriate) chart options are usually available to choose from, there is usually no single best chart for a given data set. The ideal is to consider multiple charts, but in practice people may lack the time, skill, or inclination to do so – and may opt for a single chart that suits their circumstances.

We will now consider each of the three charts in Figure 2 in more detail.

2.1.1 The Run Chart

The first chart (Figure 2, top panel) is known as a run chart.[16] The simplest form of a chart, the run chart plots the data over time with a single central line that represents the median value.

The median is a midpoint value (=174) that separates the blood pressure data into an upper and lower half. This is useful because, in the long run, the

(a)

Reading number	1	2	3	4	5	6	7	8	9	10	11	12	13
Systolic blood pressure	169	172	175	174	161	142	174	171	168	174	180	194	161

Reading number	14	15	16	17	18	19	20	21	22	23	24	25	26
Systolic blood pressure	181	175	176	186	166	157	183	177	171	185	176	181	174

Figure 2 Three types of control charts based on the blood pressure readings of a hypertensive patient. In part b, the top panel is a run chart, the middle panel is a Shewhart control chart, and the bottom panel is a cumulative sum chart

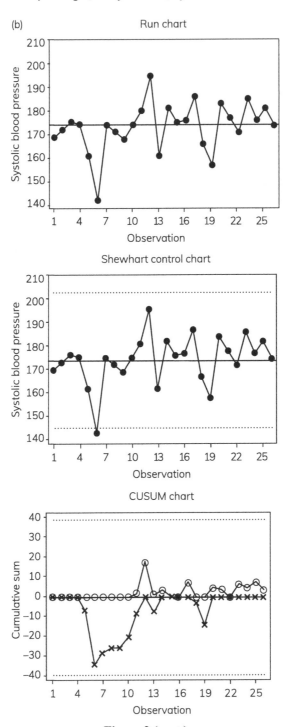

Figure 2 (cont.)

output of a stable process should appear above the median half the time and below the median the other half of the time. For example, tossing a coin would, in the long term, show heads (or tails) half the time. On a run chart, the output of a stable process will appear to bounce around the central line without unusual, non-random patterns.

The appearance of unusual (non-random) patterns would signal the presence of special cause variation. A run of six or more consecutive points above (or below) the median constitutes an unusual run, because the probability of this happening by random chance alone is less than 2% ($=0.5^6$) – for example the equivalent of tossing a coin and getting six heads in a row.

As illustrated by Figure 3, four commonly used rules[16] may detect special causes of variation with run charts (although other rules have been suggested[19,20]).

- Rule 1: A shift.
- Rule 2: A trend.
- Rule 3: Too few or too many runs above or below the median.
- Rule 4: A data point judged by eye to be unusually large or small.[16]

The run chart can be especially useful in the early stages of efforts to monitor or improve a process where there is not enough data available to reliably calculate the control limits.

When there is enough data (typically we need 20–25 data points), we can plot a Shewhart control chart (middle panel in Figure 2).[15]

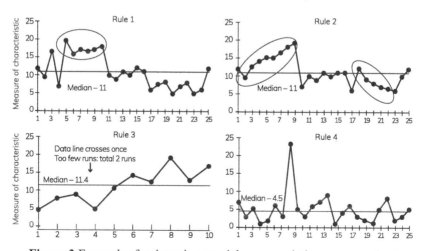

Figure 3 Four rules for detecting special cause variation on a run chart
Adapted from Perla et al.[16]

2.1.2 Shewhart Control Charts

This, like the run chart, also shows the blood pressure data over time but now with three additional lines – an average central line, and lower and upper control limits – to help identify common and special cause variation.

Data points that appear within the control limits (without any unusual patterns) are deemed to be consistent with common cause variation. Signals of special cause variation are data points that appear outside the limits or unusual patterns within the limits.

Five rules are commonly used for detecting special cause variation in a Shewhart control chart (also shown in Figure 4, enclosed by an oval shape).[15]

- Rule 1 identifies sudden changes in a process.
- Rule 2 signals smaller but sustained changes in a process.
- Rule 3 detects drift in a process.
- Rule 4 identifies more subtle runs not picked up by the other rules.
- Rule 5 identifies a process which has too little variation.

In a Shewhart control chart, the central line is usually the mean/average value. The upper and lower control limits indicate how far the data from a process can deviate from the central line based on a statistical measure of spread known as the standard deviation. Typically, about

- 60%–70% of data from a stable process will lie within ± one standard deviation of the mean.
- 90%–98% of data points lie within ± two standard deviations of the mean.
- 99%–100% of data points lie within ± three standard deviations of the mean.

Upper and lower control limits are usually set at ± three standard deviations from the mean. Setting the control limits at ± three standard deviations from the mean will capture almost all the common cause variability from a stable process. In practice, it is not uncommon to see control charts with two and three standard deviation limits shown – usually as an aid to visualisation, but also as a reminder that a judgement has to be made about where to set the limits. That judgement needs to balance the cost of looking for special cause variation when it doesn't exist against the cost of overlooking it when it does.[4,15]

It is important to understand that the variability in the data is what determines the width between the lower and upper control limits. For example, Figure 5 illustrates the impact of variability on the control limits. We see two randomly

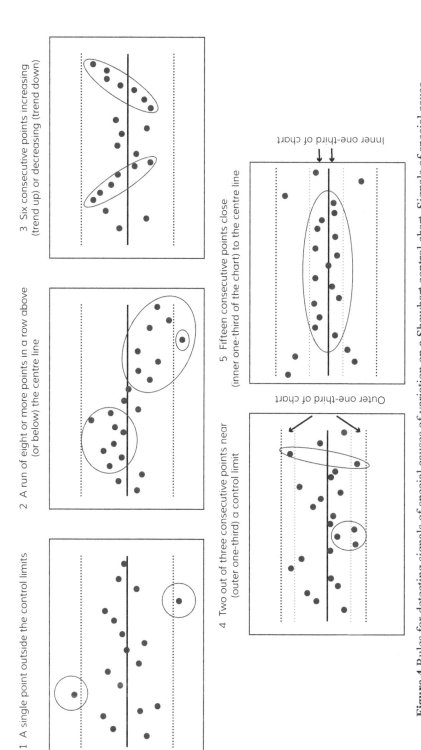

1 A single point outside the control limits

2 A run of eight or more points in a row above (or below) the centre line

3 Six consecutive points increasing (trend up) or decreasing (trend down)

4 Two out of three consecutive points near (outer one-third) a control limit

Outer one-third of chart

5 Fifteen consecutive points close (inner one-third of the chart) to the centre line

Inner one-third of chart

Figure 4 Rules for detecting signals of special causes of variation on a Shewhart control chart. Signals of special cause variation are enclosed by an oval

Adapted from Provost et al.[15]

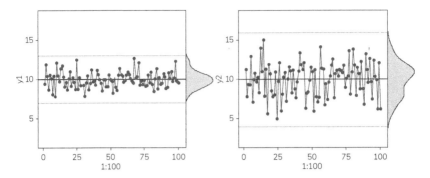

Figure 5 Control charts for two simulated random processes with identical
means (10) but the process on the right has twice the variability

generated data sets (y1 and y2) with 100 numbers having the same mean (10)
but different standard deviations (1 and 2, respectively). These data are shown
with control limits set at ± three standard deviations from the mean. The
increased variability in y2 is associated with wider control limits. Both processes are stable in that they show random variation, but the process on the right
has greater variation and hence wider control limits.

We next consider another approach to charting based on accumulating differences in the data set using CUSUM charts.

2.1.3 Cumulative Sum Charts

The bottom panel in Figure 2 shows a CUSUM chart.[18] Unlike the other two charts,
it doesn't show the raw blood pressure measurements. Instead, it shows the
differences between the raw data and a selected target (the mean in this case)
accumulated over time. For a stable process, the cumulative sums will hover around
zero (the central line is zero on a CUSUM chart), indicating common cause
variation. If the CUSUM line breaches the upper or lower control limit, this is
a sign of special cause variation, indicating that the process has drifted away from
its target.

CUSUM charts are more complex to construct and less intuitive than run charts
or Shewhart charts, but they are effective in detecting signals of special cause
variation – especially from smaller shifts in the behaviour of a process. The
CUSUM chart in Figure 2 is a two-sided CUSUM plot because it tracks deviations above and below the target. But in practice, a one-sided CUSUM plot is
often used because the primary aim is to spot an increase or decrease in performance. For example, when monitoring complication rates after surgery, the focus is
on detecting any deterioration in performance – for which a one-sided CUSUM
plot is appropriate.[21]

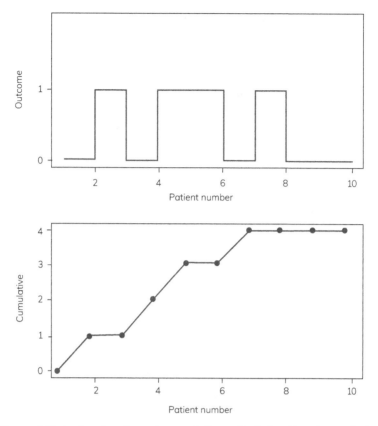

Figure 6 Plots showing the outcomes (alive = 0, died = 1) and cumulative outcomes for 10 patients following surgery

An important use for CUSUM charts in healthcare is to monitor binary outcomes on a case-by-case basis, such as post-operative outcomes (e.g. alive or died) following surgery. As an illustration, we can indicate patients who survived or died with 0 and 1, respectively. Let's say we have a sequence for 10 consecutive patients, as 0,1,0,1,1,0,1,0,0,0. Although we can plot such a sequence of 0s and 1s on a run chart or Shewhart chart, this proves to be of little use because the data steps up or down on the chart constrained at 0 or 1 (Figure 6, top panel). However, the CUSUM chart (Figure 6, bottom panel) uses these data more effectively by accumulating the sequence of 0s and 1s over time. A change in slope indicates a death, and a horizontal shift (i.e. no change in slope) indicates survival.

3 Statistical Process Control in Action

In this section, we look at how statistical process control charts are used in practice in healthcare, where they generally serve two broad purposes: (1) to monitor an existing process, or (2) as an integral part of efforts to improve a process. The two are not mutually exclusive: for example, we might begin to monitor a process and then decide that its performance is unsatisfactory and needs to be improved; once improved, we can go back to monitoring it. The following case studies show how statistical process control charts have been used in healthcare for either purpose. We begin with the run chart.

3.1 Improving Patient Flow in an Acute Hospital Using Run Charts

Run charts offer simple and intuitive ways of seeing how a process is behaving over time and assessing the impact of interventions on that process. Run charts are easy to construct (as they mainly involve plotting the data over time) and can be useful for both simple and complex interventions. This section discusses how run charts were used to support efforts to address patient flow issues in an acute hospital in England.[22]

Patients who arrive at a hospital can experience unnecessary delays because of poor patient flow, which often happens because of a mismatch between capacity and demand. No one wins from poor patient flow: it can threaten the quality and safety of care, undermine patient satisfaction and staff morale, and increase costs. Enhancing patient flow requires healthcare teams and departments across the hospital to align and synchronise to the needs of patients in a timely manner. But this is a complex challenge because it involves many stakeholders across multiple teams and departments.

A multidisciplinary team undertook a patient flow analysis focusing on older emergency patients admitted to the Geriatric Medicine Directorate of Sheffield Teaching Hospitals NHS Foundation Trust (around 920 beds).[22] The team found a mismatch between demand and capacity: 60% of older patients (aged 75+ years) were arriving in the emergency department during office hours, but two-thirds of subsequent admissions to general medical wards took place outside office hours. This highlighted a major delay between arriving at the emergency department and admission to a ward.

The team was clear that more beds was not the answer, saying that an operational strategy that seeks to increase bed stock to keep up with demand was not only financially unworkable but also 'diverts us from uncovering the shortcomings in our current systems and patterns of work'.[22]

The team used a combination of the Institute for Healthcare Improvement's Model for Improvement (which incorporates PDSA cycles – see the Element on the Institute for Healthcare Improvement approach[3]), lean methodology (a set of operating philosophies and methods that help create maximum value for patients by reducing waste and waits), and statistical process control methodology to develop and test three key changes: a discharge to assess policy, seven-day working, and the establishment of a frailty unit. Overall progress was tracked using a daily bed occupancy run chart (Figure 7) as the key analytical tool. The team annotated the chart with improvement efforts as well as other possible reasons for special cause variation, such as public holidays. This synthesis of process knowledge and patterns on the chart enabled the team to assess, in real time, the extent to which their efforts were impacting on bed occupancy. Since daily bed occupancy data are not serially independent – unlike the tossing of a coin – the team did not use the run tests associated with run charts and so based the central line on the mean, not the median.

The run chart enabled the team to see the impact of their process changes and share this with other staff. It is clear from the run chart that bed occupancy has fallen over time (Figure 7).

The team also used run charts to concurrently monitor a suite of measures (shown over four panels in Figure 8) to assess the wider impact of the changes:[22] bed occupancy, in-hospital mortality, and re-admission rates over time before and after the intervention (vertical dotted line). Bed occupancy was the key indicator of flow. In-hospital mortality was an outcome measure, while admission and re-admission to hospital were balancing measures. The latter are important because balancing measures can satisfy the need to track potential unintended consequences of healthcare improvement efforts (see the Element on the Institute for Healthcare Improvement approach[3]). Plotting this bundle as run charts alongside each other enabled visual inspection of the alignment between the measures and changes made by the team. The charts in Figure 8 show:

- a fall in bed occupancy after the intervention
- a drop in mortality after the intervention
- no change in re-admission rates
- a slight increase in the number of admissions (116.2 (standard deviation 15.7) per week before the intervention versus 122.8 (standard deviation 20.2) after).

While introducing major changes to a complex adaptive system, the team was able to use simple run charts showing a suite of related measures to inform their progress. They demonstrated how improving patient flow resulted in higher quality, lower costs, and improved working for staff: 'As a consequence of these changes, we were able to close one ward and transfer the nursing, therapy, and clerical staff to fill staff vacancies elsewhere and so reduce agency staff costs.'[22] As Perla et al. note: 'The run chart allows us to learn a great deal about the performance of our process with minimal mathematical complexity.'[16]

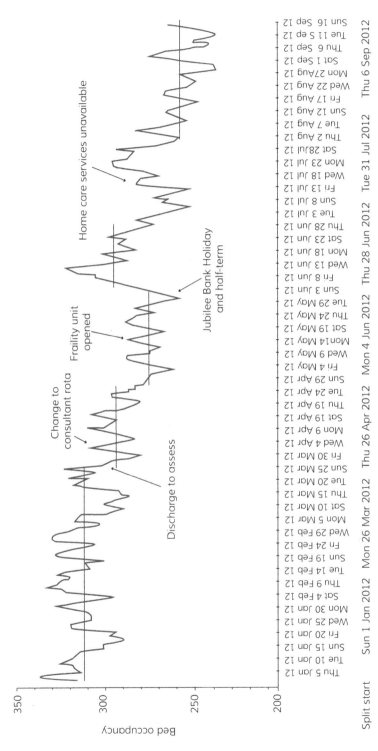

Figure 7 Daily bed occupancy run chart for geriatric medicine with annotations identifying system changes and unusual patterns

Adapted from Silvester et al.[22]

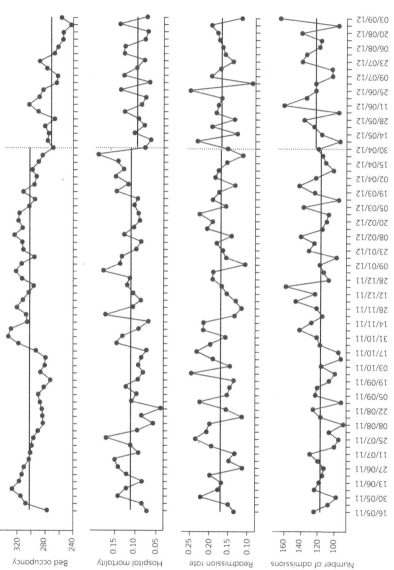

Figure 8 Run charts for bed occupancy, mortality, readmission rate, and number of admissions over time in weeks (69 weeks from 16 May 2011 to 3 September 2012) with horizontal lines indicating the mean before and after the intervention (indicated by a vertical dotted line in week 51, 30 April 2012)

Adapted from Silvester et al.[22]

The next example shows the use of control charts for managing individual patients with high blood pressure.

3.2 Managing Individual Patients with Hypertension through Use of Statistical Process Control

Chronic disease represents a major challenge to healthcare providers across the world. A crucial issue is finding ways for healthcare professionals to work in partnership with patients to better manage it. In this section, we look at a case study that shows how this was achieved using statistical process control methodology.

Hebert and Neuhauser describe a case study of a 71-year-old man with uncontrolled high blood pressure and type 2 diabetes.[23] Managing high blood pressure presents difficulties for both physicians and patients. A key challenge is obtaining meaningful measures of the level of blood pressure control and of changes in blood pressure after an intervention. In this case, the patient's mean office systolic blood pressure was 169mmHg over a three-year period (spanning 13 visits to general medical clinics) compared with the target of 130mmHg. The patient was then referred to a blood pressure clinic.

At the initial clinic visit in April 2003, the first pharmacologic intervention was offered: an increase in the dose of hydrochlorothiazide from 25mg to 50mg daily, along with advice to increase dietary potassium intake. The physician also ordered a home blood pressure monitor and gave the patient graph paper to record his blood pressure readings from home in the form of a run chart. On his second visit, the patient brought his run chart of 30 home blood pressure readings. The physician later plotted these data on a Shewhart control chart (Figure 9, left panel). The mean systolic blood pressure fell to 131.1mmHg (target 130mmHg), with upper and lower control limits of 146mmHg and 116mmHg, respectively. The patient agreed to continue recording his blood pressure and returned for a third visit in September 2003. Figure 9 (right panel) shows these blood pressure observations with a reduced mean value of 126.1mmHg, which is below the target value with no obvious special cause variation.

The perspectives of both patient and physician are recorded in Box 2, which highlight how partnership working was enhanced by the use of control charts.

A systematic review of statistical process control methods in monitoring clinical variables in individual patients reports that they are used across a range of conditions – high blood pressure, asthma, renal function post-transplant, and diabetes.[7] The review concludes that statistical process control charts appear to have a promising but largely under-researched role in

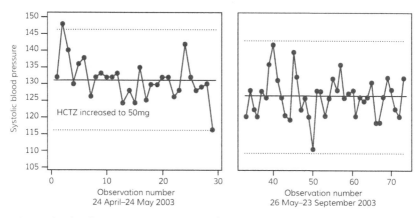

Figure 9 Blood pressure control charts between two consecutive clinic visits
Adapted from Herbert and Neuhauser[23]

monitoring clinical variables in individual patients; the review calls for more rigorous evaluation of their use.

The next example shows the use of statistical process methods to monitor the performance of individual surgeons.

3.3 Monitoring the Performance of Individual Surgeons through CUSUM Charts

The Scottish Arthroplasty Project aims for continual improvement in the quality of care provided to patients undergoing a joint replacement in Scotland.[24] Supported by the Chief Medical Officer for Scotland and wholly funded by the Scottish government, the project is led by orthopaedic surgeons and reports to the Scottish Committee for Orthopaedics and Trauma. Its steering committee includes orthopaedic surgeons, an anaesthetist, patient representatives, and community medicine representatives. Scotland has a population of 5.2 million and is served by 24 orthopaedic National Health Service (NHS) provider units with about 300 surgeons.

The project analyses the performance of individual consultant surgeons based on five routinely collected outcome measures: death, dislocation, wound infection, revision arthroplasty, and venous thromboembolism. Every three months, each surgeon is provided with a personalised report detailing the outcomes of all their operations.

Outcomes are monitored using CUSUM charts, which are well suited to monitoring adverse events per operation for individual surgeons while also accounting for the differences in risk between patients. Figure 10 shows three examples of CUSUM charts.

BOX 2 A PATIENT'S AND A PHYSICIAN'S PERSPECTIVES ON USING CONTROL CHARTS[23]

The Patient's Perspective	The Physician's Perspective

I enjoyed plotting my readings and being able to clearly see that I was making progress. The activity takes about 10 minutes out of my day, which is only a minor inconvenience. After several weeks of recording daily readings, I settled on readings approximately three times a week. After five months, I think this is an activity that I will be able to continue indefinitely. I feel that my target blood pressure has been met because the systolic blood pressure is generally below 130mmHg. Since I began this activity I have a good idea of the status of my blood pressure, whereas prior to starting, I had only a vague idea, which bothered me. Occasionally, a reading would be unusually high, for example 142. In such cases, I worried that the device may not be working, and I would check my wife's blood pressure. She too has high blood pressure, and if her reading was close to her typical pressure, I would say that my own pressure really was high that day. I would not change what I do because of a single high reading and I would not be alarmed. If my pressure was more than 130mmHg for a week or so then I'd probably call the doctor.

My job was made easier by the presence of a continuous stream of data. I was able to learn with a fair degree of certainty that the intervention was effective at lowering blood pressure, and if the level of elevated blood pressure persists, then the intervention should lower cardiovascular risk. ... I have preliminary data on the 33 patients in our clinic with high blood pressure, who have follow-up data to compare baseline and current blood pressure. This group consists exclusively of patients with a history of poorly controlled blood pressure. Of the 33 patients, 31 have lowered their blood pressure, by a mean of 20 points.

Of these patients, 22 are presently keeping run charts and periodically bringing them back to the office, whereas the others are more comfortable with recording the values in tabular form. A few were initially uncomfortable with graphing, but then began after seeing copies of run charts created by their peers in the programme. Among the patients using run charts, a consistent message is that it is not a burden, and furthermore many have expressed the opinion that it is an enlightening activity.

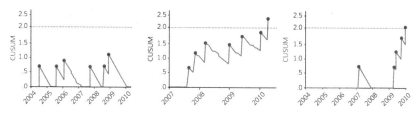

Figure 10 Example CUSUM charts for three surgeons

Adapted from Macpherson et al.[24]

- The left panel is a CUSUM chart for a surgeon who operated from 2004 to 2010. Each successful operation is shown as a grey dot; each operation with a complication is shown as a black dot. The CUSUM rises if there is a complication and falls if there is not. The CUSUM for this surgeon remains stable, indicating common cause variation.
- The middle panel shows a surgeon with a rising CUSUM mostly above zero – indicating a consistently higher-than-average complication rate. In 2010, the upper control limit is breached triggering a signal of special cause variation that merits investigation.
- The right panel shows a CUSUM chart that is unremarkable until 2009 but suggests a possible change to the underlying process thereafter, such as a new technique or new implant, for example.

Because complications are rare events, they cause a large rise in the CUSUM, whereas multiple operations that have no complication will each cause a small decrease in the CUSUM. The two will therefore tend to cancel each other out, and if a surgeon's complication rate is close to or below average, their CUSUM will hover not far from zero. On the other hand, a surgeon who has an unusually high number of complications will have a CUSUM that exceeds the horizontal control limit. Such a surgeon is labelled an 'outlier' in the Scottish Arthroplasty Project.

The value of the horizontal control limit line (in this case 2) is a management decision based on a judgement that balances the risks of false alerts (occurring by chance when the surgeon's complication rate is in control), and the risk of not detecting an unacceptable change in complication rate. The project team chose a control limit of 2 because it allows detection of special cause variation for as few as four complications in quick succession.

This CUSUM-based monitoring scheme is part of a comprehensive data collection, analysis, and feedback system focusing on individual surgeons (see Figure 11). If a CUSUM plot for an individual surgeon exceeds the horizontal dotted line (Figure 10), the surgeon will be alerted, asked to review their complications and to complete and return an action plan to the project steering committee (see Figure 11).

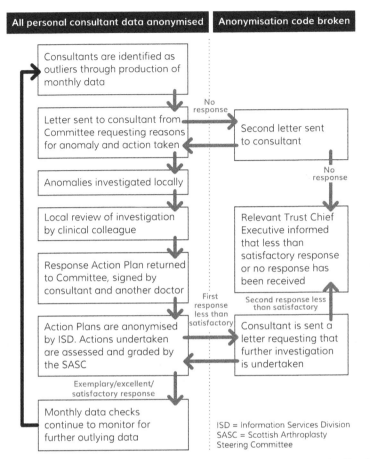

Figure 11 Flowchart showing the process of data collection and feedback
Adapted from Macpherson et al.[24]

A major advantage of this CUSUM scheme is that it identifies signals quickly because the analysis shows the outcome of each operation. This allows for the rapid identification of failing implants or poor practices and allows implants to be withdrawn or practices to be changed in a timely manner.

The CUSUM chart is reset to zero once the project steering committee receives an explanation from the surgeon involved. A comprehensive case note review reflecting a difficult casemix can also form the basis of a constructive response. Responses are graded into one of four categories, as shown in the table in Figure 12. The chart in Figure 12 shows how responses have changed over time. The authors note: 'As surgeons have become more aware of the feedback system, particularly with the introduction of CUSUM, their responses have become more rapid and more comprehensive.'[24]

Action Plan Outcomes	
Exemplary	Constructive response with evidence of progress
Excellent	Constructive response
Satisfactory	Minimum requirement
Less than satisfactory	Unacceptable

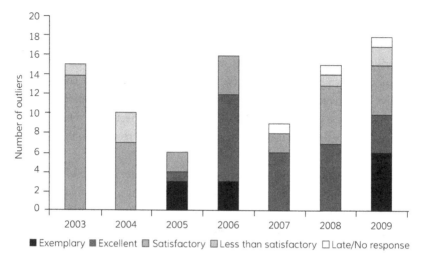

Figure 12 Table and accompanying graph showing how action plans were graded

Adapted from Macpherson et al.[24]

The authors report that

> *[w]ithin the Scottish orthopaedic community, there has been a general accept-ance of the role of Scottish Arthroplasty Project as an independent clinical governance process. From surgeons' feedback, we know that notification of an outlying position presents a good opportunity for self-review even if no obvious problems are identified. When local management has questioned individual practice, Scottish Arthroplasty Project data are made available to the surgeon to support the surgeon's practice. This type of data has also been valuable in appraisal processes that will feed into the future professional revalidation system. Data also can be useful to the surgeon in medical negligence cases. Although there were initially concerns about lack of engagement from the orthopaedic surgeons, our methodology has resulted in enthusiasm from the surgeons and 100% compliance. We have found that the process has nurtured innovation, education, and appropriate risk aversion.*[24]

The next example is a landmark study that showed how statistical process control supported reductions in complications following surgery in France.

3.4 Reducing Complications after Surgery Using Statistical Process Control

Healthcare-related adverse events are a major cause of illness and death. Around 1 in 10 patients who undergo surgery are estimated to experience a preventable complication.[25] In a landmark randomised controlled trial, a multidisciplinary team from France investigated the extent to which major adverse patient events were reduced by using statistical process control charts to monitor post-surgery outcomes and feed the data back to surgical teams.[25]

Duclos et al. randomised 40 hospitals to either usual care (control hospitals) or to quarterly control charts (intervention hospitals) monitoring four patient-focused outcomes following digestive surgery: inpatient death, unplanned admission to intensive care, reoperation, and a combination of severe complications (cardiac arrest, pulmonary embolism, sepsis, or surgical site infection).[25] Our focus is primarily on how the team used statistical process control methods in the intervention hospitals.

P-charts (where p stands for proportion or percentage) are useful for monitoring binary outcomes (e.g. alive, died) as a percentage over time (e.g. percentage of patients who died following surgery).[26] The 20 intervention hospitals used a p-control chart to monitor the four outcomes (example in Figure 13). The charts included three and two standard deviation control limits set around the central line. A signal of special cause variation was defined as a single point outside the three standard deviation control limit or two of three successive points outside the two standard deviation limits.

The authors recognised that successful implementation of control charts in healthcare required a leadership culture that allowed staff to learn from variation by investigating special causes of variation and trying out and evaluating quality improvement initiatives.[25] To enable successful implementation of the control chart, 'champion partnerships' were established at each site, comprising a surgeon and another member of the surgical team (surgeon, anaesthetist, or nurse).[25] Each duo was responsible for conducting meetings to review the control chart and keeping a logbook in which changes in care processes were recorded. Champion partners from each hospital met at three one-day training sessions held at eight-month intervals. Simulated role-play at these sessions aimed to provide the skills needed to use the control charts appropriately, lead review meetings for effective cooperation and decision-making, identify variations in special causes, and devise plans for improvement.

Over two years post-intervention, the control charts were analysed at perioperative team meetings.[25] Unfavourable signals of special cause variation triggered examination of potential causes, which led to an average of 20 changes for each

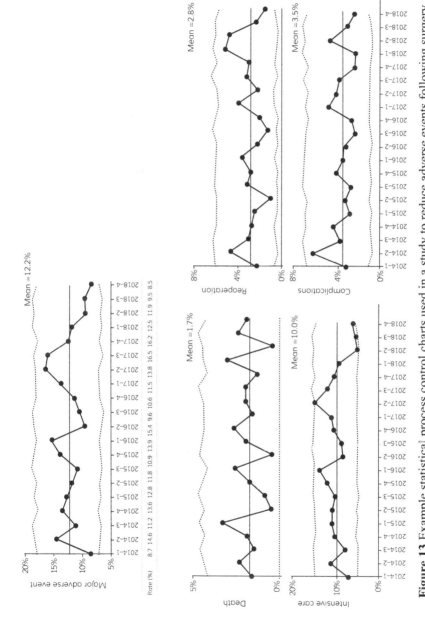

Figure 13 Example statistical process control charts used in a study to reduce adverse events following surgery

Adapted from Duclos et al.[25]

Hospital number	1	2	3	4	5	6	7	8	9	10	11	12	13	14	15	16	17	18	19	20	Total
Duo formed with a surgeon	1	1	1	1	1	1	1	1	1	1	1	1	1	1	1	1	1	1	1	1	20
Participation in all three training sessions	1	1	1	1	1	1	1	1	1	1	1	1	1	1	1	1	1		1		18
Logbook updated until the end	1	1	1	1	1	1	1	1	1	1											9
Eight posters displayed in operating room	1	1	1	1	1				1									1			7
Eight team team meetings held	1	1	1	1	1	1	1	1	1	1	1	1									12
At least one improvement action tested	1	1	1	1	1	1	1	1	1	1	1	1	1	1	1	1	1	1		1	19
Implementation score	6	6	6	6	6	5	5	5	5	4	4	4	4	4	4	4	3	3	2	2	4.3
Compliance degree	High									Moderate									Poor		

Figure 14 Compliance of hospitals in the intervention arm using control charts *Adapted from Duclos et al.*[25]

intervention hospital (Figure 14). Compared with the control hospitals, the intervention hospitals recorded significant reductions in rates of major adverse events (a composite of all outcome indicators). The absolute risk of a major adverse event was reduced by 0.9% in intervention compared with control hospitals – this equates to one major adverse event prevented for every 114 patients treated in hospitals using the quarterly control charts.[25] Among the intervention hospitals, the size of the effect was proportional to the degree of control chart implementation. Duclos et al. conclude: 'The value of control charts and sharing ideas within surgical teams designed to eliminate patient harm has been mostly underappreciated.'[25]

The next example shows the use of statistical process control to compare the performance of healthcare organisations.

3.5 Comparing the Performance of Healthcare Organisations Using Funnel Plots

Monitoring of healthcare organisations is now ubiquitous.[27] Comparing organisations has often taken the form of performance league tables (also known as caterpillar plots – see Figure 15a), which rank providers according to a performance metric such as mortality. Such tables have been criticised for focusing on spurious rankings that fail to distinguish between common and special causes of variation.[28] Despite these concerns, they were widely used to compare the performance of provider units until the introduction of statistical process control-based funnel plots[27] (see Figure 15b: here, the funnel plot has two sets of control limits corresponding to two and three standard deviations).

The funnel plot is a scatter graph of the metric of interest (post-operative mortality in Figure 15) on the y-axis versus the number of cases (sample size) on the x-axis across a group of healthcare organisations. Such data are cross-sectional (not over time), so there is no time dimension to the funnel plot. The funnel plot takes a process or systems perspective by showing upper and lower control limits around the overall mean instead of individual limits around each hospital (as shown in the caterpillar plot).

(a)

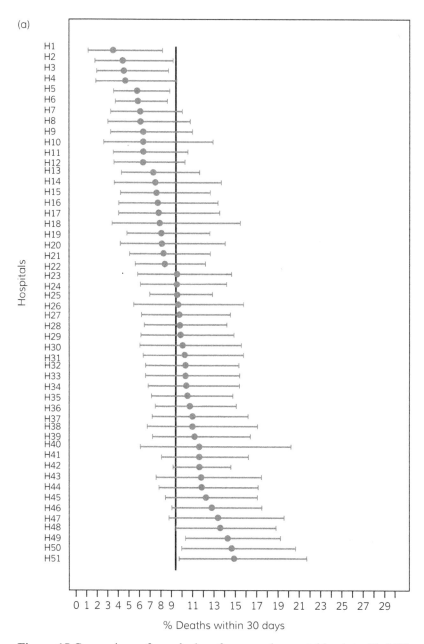

Figure 15 Comparison of a ranked performance league table plot with 95% confidence intervals (part a) versus a funnel plot with 3 sigma control limits (part b)

Adapted from Spigelhalter[27]

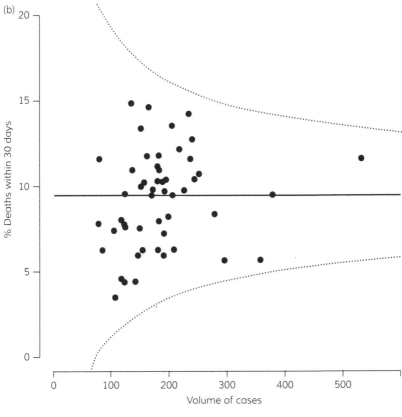

Figure 15 (cont.)

An attractive feature of the funnel plot is that the control limits get narrower as sample sizes increase. This produces the funnel shape that shows how common cause variability reduces with respect to the number of cases (the so-called outcome-volume effect). It makes it very clear that smaller units show greater common cause variation compared to larger units.

Funnel plots are now widely used for comparing performance between health-care organisations.[29–31] Spiegelhalter gives a comprehensive explanation of funnel plots for institutional comparisons,[27] and Verburg et al. provide step-by-step guidelines on the use of funnel plots in practice (based on the Dutch National Intensive Care Evaluation registry).[29] Steps include selection of the quality metric of interest, examining whether the number of observations per hospital is sufficient, and specifying how the funnel plot should be constructed.

Guthrie et al.[30] show how funnel plots can be used to compare the performance of general practices across a range of performance indicators. In Figure 16, the left panel shows a funnel plot for one performance indicator over all the

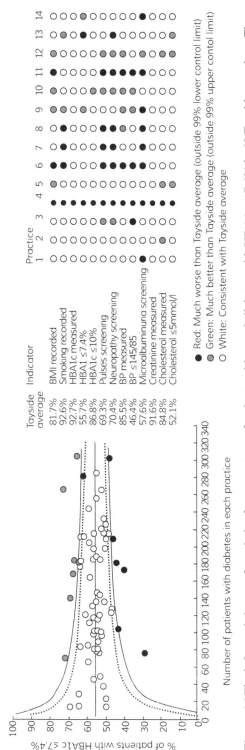

Practice 1 2 3 4 5 6 7 8 9 10 11 12 13 14

Indicator	Tayside average
BMI recorded	81.7%
Smoking recorded	92.6%
HBA1c measured	92.7%
HBA1 ≤7.4%	55.7%
HBA1c ≤10%	86.8%
Pulses screening	69.3%
Neuropathy screening	70.4%
BP measured	85.5%
BP ≤145/85	46.4%
Microalbuminuria screening	57.6%
Creatinine measured	91.6%
Cholesterol measured	84.8%
Cholesterol ≤5mmol/l	52.1%

● Red: Much worse than Tayside average (outside 99% lower control limit)
◉ Green: Much better than Tayside average (outside 99% upper contol limit)
○ White: Consistent with Tayside average

% of patients with HBA1C ≤7.4%

0 20 40 60 80 100 120 140 160 180 200 220 240 260 280 300 320 340

Number of patients with diabetes in each practice

Figure 16 The left panel shows a funnel plot for percentage of patients with type 2 diabetes with HBA1c ≤7.4% in 69 Tayside practices. The right panel summarises the signals from 13 other performance indicator funnel plots across 14 general practices

Adapted from Guthrie et al.[30]

practices in Tayside, Scotland. The right panel shows a statistical process control dashboard for 13 performance indicators across 14 practices. The use of red-white-green categories should not be confused with the usual red-amber-green (RAG) reporting seen in hospital performance reports;[32] the former is based on statistical process control methodology, and the latter is not.

Although funnel plots do not show the behaviour of a process over time, they can still be used to compare performance across time periods through a sequence of funnel plots. This can be illustrated using data from a public inquiry established in 1998 to probe high death rates following paediatric cardiac surgery at Bristol Royal Infirmary.[33] The data included a comparison of death rates of children under 1 year of age with data from 11 other hospitals where paediatric cardiac surgery took place. Comparisons were presented over three time periods: 1984–87, 1988–90, and 1991–March 95. Figure 17 shows this data as side-by-side funnel plots.

Bristol (centre 1) exhibits a signal of special cause variation in the third epoch (time period) only. The factors that contributed to the high death rates at Bristol were subject to a lengthy inquiry (1998–2001), which identified a range of issues.[33] A closer look at all three panels suggests Bristol's death rate stood still, whereas all other centres experienced reduced mortality. Although external action to address concerns about paediatric cardiac surgery at Bristol Royal Infirmary took place in 1998, monitoring using control charts might have provoked action earlier, in 1987.

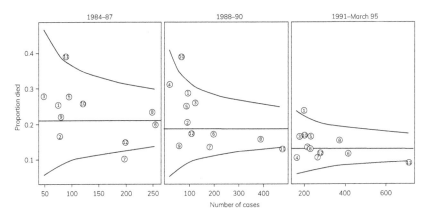

Figure 17 The Bristol data, showing mortality following cardiac surgery in children under 1 year of age. Each panel of the figure shows a control chart for the three epochs (panels, left to right: 1984–87, 1988–90, and 1991–March 95). The numbers in the panel indicate centres (1–12), the horizontal line is the mean for that epoch, and the solid lines represent three-sigma upper and lower control limits. Bristol (centre 1) clearly shows special cause variation in the third time period (1991–95) as it appears above the upper control limit

The control chart usefully guides attention to high-mortality centres (above the upper control limit), but it also identifies opportunities for improvement by learning from centres with particularly low death rates (those below the lower control limit). For example, centre 11 appears to have made remarkable reductions in mortality over the three epochs. This clearly merits investigation and, if appropriate, dissemination of practices to other hospitals.

Statistical process control methodology, then, offers an approach to learning from both favourable (see the Element on positive deviance[2]) and unfavourable signals of special causes of variation. So, how might we systematically investigate signals of special cause variation?

3.6 Investigating Special Cause Variation in Healthcare Using the Pyramid Model

The key aim of using statistical process control charts to monitor healthcare processes is to ensure that quality and safety of care are adequate and not deteriorating. When a signal of special cause variation is seen on a control chart monitoring a given outcome (e.g. mortality rates following surgery), investigation is necessary. However, the chosen method must recognise that the link between recorded outcomes and quality of care is complex, ambiguous, and subject to multiple explanations.[34] Failure to do so may inadvertently contribute to premature conclusions and a blame culture that undermines the engagement of clinical staff and the credibility of statistical process control. As Rogers et al. note: "If monitoring schemes are to be accepted by those whose outcomes are being assessed, an atmosphere of constructive evaluation, not 'blaming' or 'naming and shaming', is essential as apparent poor performance could arise for a number of reasons that should be explored systematically."[21]

To address this need, Mohammed et al. propose the Pyramid Model for Investigating Special Cause Variation in Healthcare[35] (Figure 18)[36] – a systematic approach of hypothesis generation and testing based on five theoretical candidate explanations for special cause variation: data, patient casemix, structure or resources, process of care, and carer(s).

These broad categories of candidate explanations are arranged from most likely (data) to least likely (carers), so offering a road map for the investigation that begins at the base of the pyramid and stops at the level that provides a credible, evidence-based explanation for the special cause. The first two layers of the model (data and casemix factors) provide a check on the validity of the data and casemix-adjusted analyses, whereas the remaining upper layers focus more on quality of care-related issues.

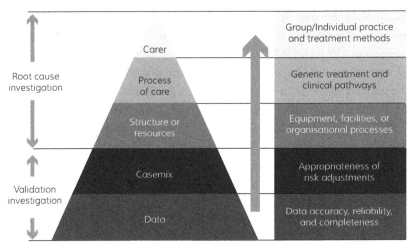

Figure 18 The Pyramid Model for investigating special cause variation in healthcare

Adapted from Mohammed et al.[35] and Smith et al.[36]

BOX 3 THE THREE BASIC STEPS FOR USING THE PYRAMID MODEL TO INVESTIGATE SPECIAL CAUSE VARIATION IN HEALTHCARE

1. Form a multidisciplinary team that has expertise in each layer of the pyramid, with a decision-making process that allows them to judge the extent to which a credible cause or explanation has been found, based on hypothesis generation and testing.
2. Candidate hypotheses are generated and tested starting from the lowest level of the Pyramid Model and proceeding to upper levels only if the preceding levels provide no adequate explanation for the special cause.
3. A credible cause requires quantitative and qualitative evidence, which is used by the team to test hypotheses and reach closure. If no credible explanation can be found, then the most likely explanation is that the signal itself was a false signal.

A proper investigation requires a team of people with expertise in each of the layers. Such a team is also likely to include those staff whose outcomes or data are being investigated, so that their insights and expertise can inform the investigation while also ensuring their buy-in to the investigation process. Basic steps for using the model are shown in Box 3.

Mohammed et al. first demonstrated the use of the Pyramid Model to identify a credible explanation for the high mortality associated with two general practitioners (GPs) flagged by the Shipman Inquiry. Their mortality data showed evidence of special cause variation on risk-adjusted CUSUM charts (see Box 4).[35]

BOX 4 THE USE OF THE PYRAMID MODEL TO INVESTIGATE HIGH-MORTALITY GENERAL
PRACTITIONERS FLAGGED UP BY THE SHIPMAN INQUIRY

Harold Shipman (1946–2004) was an English GP who is believed to be the most prolific serial killer in history. In January 2000, a jury found Shipman guilty of the murder of 15 patients under his care, with his total number of victims estimated to be around 250. A subsequent high-profile public inquiry included an analysis of mortality data involving a sample of 1,009 GPs. Using CUSUM plots, the analysis highlighted 12 GPs as having high (special cause variation) patient mortality that merited investigation. One was Shipman.

Mohammed et al.[34] used the Pyramid Model to investigate the reasons behind the findings in relation to two of the GPs. They assembled a multidisciplinary team which began by checking the data. Once the data was considered to be accurate, the team had preliminary discussions with the two GPs to generate candidate hypotheses. This process highlighted deaths in nursing homes as a possible explanatory factor.

This hypothesis was tested quantitatively and qualitatively. The magnitude and shape of the curves of a CUSUM plot for excess number of deaths in each year were closely mirrored by the magnitude and shape of the curves of the number of patients dying in nursing homes; and this was reflected in the high correlations between excess mortality and the number of deaths in nursing homes in each year for the GPs. These findings were supported by administrative data. Furthermore, it was known that the casemix adjustment scheme used for the CUSUM plots did not include the place of death.

The investigation concluded: "The excessively high mortality associated with two general practitioners was credibly explained by a nursing home effect. General practitioners associated with high patient mortality, albeit after sophisticated statistical analysis, should not be labelled as having poor performance but instead should be considered as a signal meriting scientific investigation."[34]

The Pyramid Model has been incorporated into statistical process control-based monitoring schemes in Northern Ireland[37] and Queensland, Australia.[36,38] In Queensland, clinical governance arrangements now include the use of CUSUM-type statistical process control charts (known as variable life-adjusted display plots) to monitor care outcomes in 87 hospitals using 31 clinical indicators (e.g. stroke, colorectal cancer surgery, depression) derived from routinely collected data.[38] Crucially, monitoring is tied in with an approach to investigation, learning, and action that incorporates the Pyramid Model as shown in Table 1.

The next example shows how statistical process control methods were used to modify performance data in hospital board reports.

3.7 Control Charts in Hospital Board Reports

Hospital board members have to deal with large amounts of data related to quality and safety, usually in the form of hospital board reports.[39] Board members need to look at reports in detail to help identify problems with care and assure quality. However, the task is not straightforward because members need to understand the role of chance (or common cause variation) and be able to distinguish signals from noise.

In 2016, Schmidtke et al.[39] reviewed board reports for 30 randomly selected English NHS trusts (*n* = 163) and found that only 6% of the charts (*n* = 1,488) illustrated the role of chance. The left panel in Figure 19 shows an example chart which displays the number of unplanned re-admissions within 48 hours of discharge but provides no indication that chance played a role. The right panel shows a control chart of the same data but also indicates the role of chance with the aid of control limits around a central line.

Schmidtke et al. conclude: 'Control charts can help board members distinguish signals from noise, but often boards are not using them.'[39] They assumed that members might not be requesting control charts because

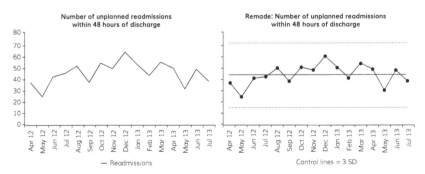

Figure 19 Example chart from a hospital board report (left) represented as a control chart (right)

Adapted from Schmidtke et al.[39]

Table 1 Use of the Pyramid Model to investigate special cause variation in hospitals in Queensland, Australia

Level	Scope	Typical Questions
Data	Data quality issues (e.g. coding accuracy, reliability of charts, definitions, and completeness)	Are the data coded correctly? Has there been a change in data coding practices (e.g. are there less experienced coders)? Is clinical documentation clear, complete, and consistent?
Casemix	Although differences in casemix are accounted for in the calculation, it is possible that some residual confounding may remain	Are there factors peculiar to this hospital not considered in the risk adjustment? Has the pattern of referrals to this hospital changed (in a way not considered in risk adjustment)?
Structure or resource	Availability of beds, staff, and medical equipment; institutional processes	Has there been a change in the distribution of patients in the hospital, with more patients in this specialty spread throughout the hospital rather than concentrated in a particular unit?
Process of care	Medical treatments of patients, clinical pathways, patient admission and discharge hospital policies	Has there been a change in the care being provided? Have new treatment guidelines been introduced?
Professional staff/ carers	Practice and treatment methods, and so on	Has there been a change in staffing for treatment of patients? Has a key staff member gained additional training and introduced a new method that has led to improved outcomes?

Adapted from Duckett et al.[38]

they were unaware of statistical process control methodology, so they suggested an active training programme for board members. And, since hospital data analysts might not have the necessary skills to produce control charts, they also proposed training for analysts. As a realistic default recommendation, they suggested using a single chart that has proven robust for most time-series data – the individuals or XmR chart. This is a useful chart, but there is controversy about its use across the different types of data in hospital board reports such as percentage data for which a p-chart is recommended (as shown in Section 3.4).[15,26,40]

In response, Riley et al.[32] devised a training programme – called Making Data Count – for board members in English NHS trusts and developed a spreadsheet tool to allow analysts to readily produce control charts. A 90-minute board training session on the use of statistical process control was delivered to 583 participants from 61 NHS trust boards between November 2017 and July 2019. Feedback from participants was that 99% of respondents felt the training session had been a good use of their time, and 97% agreed that it would enhance their ability to make good decisions. A key feature of the whole-board training programme was using hospitals' own performance data (from their board reports) to demonstrate the advantages

Figure 20 Example chart from a hospital board report (upper panel) which is underpinned by multiple statistical process control charts (lower panel)[41]

Adapted from East London NHS Foundation Trust. Board of Directors Meeting in Public. Thursday 30 March 2023.[41]

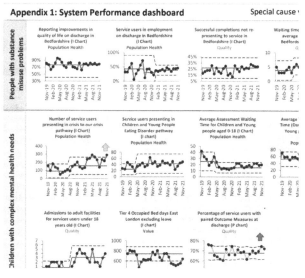

Figure 20 (cont.)

of statistical process control. Participants highlighted this in evaluation interviews (see Box 5).

Figure 20 shows an extract from a board report with an overview performance summary (upper panel) based on a multiple statistical process control chart (lower panel).

Our next example shows the use of statistical process control during the COVID-19 pandemic.

3.8 Tracking Deaths during the COVID-19 Pandemic through Shewhart Control Charts

The COVID-19 pandemic, which was declared in March 2020, has posed unprecedented challenges to healthcare systems worldwide. The daily number of deaths was a key metric of interest. Perla et al. developed a novel hybrid Shewhart chart to visualise and learn from daily variations in reported deaths. They note: "We know that the number of reported deaths each day – as with anything we measure – will fluctuate. Without a method to understand if these 'ups and downs' simply reflect natural variability, we will struggle to recognize signals of meaningful improvement . . . in epidemic conditions."[42]

Figure 21 shows a chart of daily deaths annotated with sample media headlines. It highlights how headline writers struggled to separate meaningful signals from noise in the context of a pandemic and the risk that the data might provoke 'hyperreactive responses from policy-makers and public citizens alike'.[42]

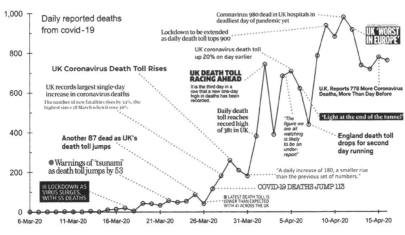

Figure 21 Headlines associated with daily reported deaths in the United Kingdom during the COVID-19 pandemic

Reproduced from Perla et al.[42]

BOX 5 THREE BOARD MEMBERS' PERSPECTIVES ON CONTROL CHARTS

The most powerful intervention was to use our own data and play it back to us. It helped us to see what's missing.

By exposing the full board to Statistical Process Control (SPC) as a way to look at measures, the training helped us all learn together and have the same level of knowledge. We all gained new insights, and it has helped us to think about where and how to begin experimenting with presenting metrics in SPC format. I thought it was terrific. In fact, I wrote a note to the chairperson to share my observation that it was the best board session I had attended in 4 years. The reason was that the training was accessible, not too basic but not too advanced; it was not too short or too long in length; and it was directly relevant and applicable to the organisation as a whole and also useful for my role.

We are already seeing changes. We have completely overhauled the board report. The contrast from July is that by September, we can see SPC in every individual section. It's made it easier to go through the board paper, and it's now significantly clearer about what we should focus on. We also chose to bring in the performance team. We wanted to get a collective understanding of what was needed. So, it was not an isolationist session; it was leaders and people who knew about the data. We wanted everyone to leave the session knowing what we were aiming for, what to do and how. There have been no additional costs. All the changes have been possible within current resources. This is about doing things in a different way. We were lucky that we had staff with good analytical skills and they have been able to do this work quickly and effectively.

Reproduced from Riley et al.[32]

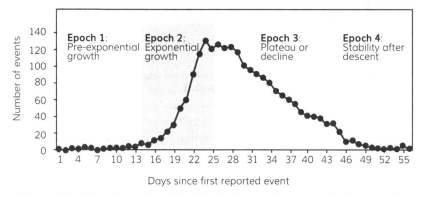

Figure 22 A hypothetical epidemiological curve for events in four epochs
Adapted from Parry et al. [43]

BOX 6 THE FOUR EPOCHS OF AN EPIDEMIC CURVE [43]

- Epoch 1 'pre-exponential growth' begins with the first reported daily event. Daily counts usually remain relatively low and stable with no evidence of exponential growth. Epoch 1 ends when rapid growth in events starts to occur and the chart moves into Epoch 2.
- Epoch 2 'exponential growth' is when daily events begin to grow rapidly. This can be alarming for those reading the chart or experiencing the pandemic. Epoch 2 ends when events start to level off (plateau) or decline.
- Epoch 3 'plateau or descent' is when daily events stop increasing exponentially. Instead, they start to 'plateau or descend'. Epoch 3 can end when daily values start to return to pre-exponential growth values. More troublingly, it can also end with a return to exponential growth (Epoch 2) – a sign that the pandemic is taking a turn for the worse again.
- Epoch 4 'stability after descent' is similar to Epoch 1 (pre-exponential growth), when a descent in daily events has occurred and daily counts are again low and stable. Epoch 4 can end if further signs of trouble are detected and there is a return to exponential growth (Epoch 2).

Using the hybrid chart, the researchers identified four phases (or 'epochs') of the classical infectious disease curve.[42,43] The four epochs are shown in Figure 22 and described in Box 6. The researchers used a combination of Shewhart control charts to track the pandemic and help separate signals (of change) from background noise in each phase.

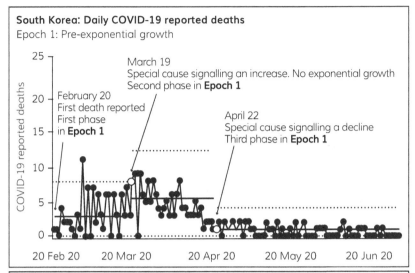

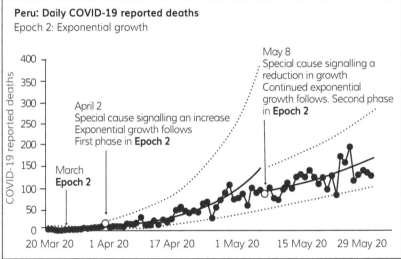

Figure 23 Shewhart charts for the four epochs of daily reported COVID-19 deaths in different countries

Adapted from Parry et al.[43]

Figure 23 shows these epochs using data from different countries; Figure 24 shows the hybrid Shewhart chart for the United Kingdom. Parry et al. state:

"Shewhart charts should be a standard tool to learn from variation in data during an epidemic. Medical professionals, improvement leaders, health officials and the public could use this chart with reported epidemic

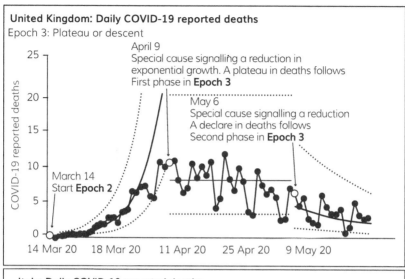

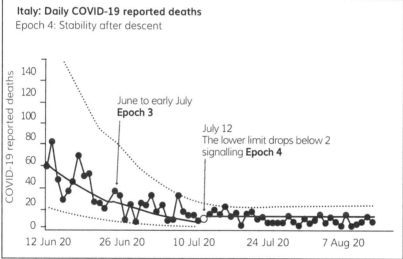

Figure 23 (cont.)

measures such as cases, testing rates, hospitalizations, intubations, and deaths to rapidly detect meaningful changes over time."[43]

The previous case studies have demonstrated the use of statistical process control methods in healthcare across a wide range of applications. In the next section, we offer a more critical examination of the methodology to identify and address the barriers to successful use in practice.

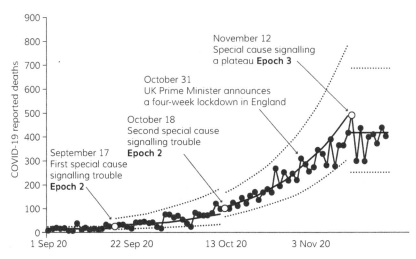

Figure 24 Hybrid Shewhart control chart for monitoring daily COVID-19 deaths in the United Kingdom

Adapted from Parry et al.[43]

4 Critiques of Statistical Process Control

Although statistical process control methodology is now widely used to monitor and improve the quality and safety of healthcare, in this section, we consider the strengths, limitations, and future role of the methodology in healthcare.

4.1 The Statistical Process Control Paradox: It's Easy Yet Not So Easy

As the case studies discussed in Section 3 show, statistical process control is not simply a graphical tool. Rather, it is a way of thinking scientifically about monitoring and improving the quality and safety of care. But while the idea of common versus special cause variation is intuitive, the successful application of statistical process control is not as easy as it might first appear, especially in complex adaptive systems like healthcare.[12] Successfully using statistical process control in healthcare usually depends on several factors, which include engaging the stakeholders; forming a team; defining the aim; selecting the process of interest; defining the metrics of interest; ensuring that data can be reliably measured, collected, fed back, and understood; and establishing baseline performance – all in a culture of continual learning and improvement. Several systematic reviews of the use of statistical process control in healthcare provide critical insights into the benefits, limitations, barriers, and facilitators to successful application.[11,12,44] Some key lessons are shown in Table 2.

Table 2 Some key lessons from systematic reviews of statistical process control in healthcare

Benefits	• Statistical process control is a simple, relatively low-cost approach that facilitates process improvement and can be applied to a wide range of processes
	• It is useful for the management of healthcare, for assessment of the learning curve, and management of individual patients
	• It can enhance engagement of different stakeholders, including patients
Limitations	• Presenting data as a statistical process control chart does not automatically lead to improvements
	• A process that is in statistical control is not necessarily clinically acceptable or adequate
	• The correct application of statistical process control requires technical skills
Barriers	• Statistical process control can sometimes meet resistance because it may imply a change of thinking and approach
	• Lack of access to reliable data and adequate IT infrastructure to support the use of statistical process control can hinder application in practice
	• Data collection and analysis for statistical process control can be time-consuming
Facilitators	• Training users in statistical process control methodology and ensuring expert technical support is available can facilitate successful application
	• Development of easy-to-use IT tools for data management and statistical process control charting can also help
	• Focusing statistical process control on clinical topics can capture the interest of clinicians

A further challenge is that statistical process control charts are not necessarily easy to build. Even when using a run chart, for example, practitioners face differing advice on how to interpret them. Three sets of run chart rules – the Anhoej, Perla, and Carey rules – have been published, but they differ significantly in their sensitivity and specificity to detecting special causes of variation,[19,20] and there is little practical guidance on how to proceed. So perhaps it is not surprising that the literature features multiple examples of technical errors. After examining 64 statistical process control charts, Koetsier et al.[44] report that almost half (48.4%) used insufficient data points, 43.7% did not transform skewed data, and 14% did not report the rules for identifying special causes of variation. The authors conclude that many published studies did not follow all methodological criteria and so increased the risk of drawing incorrect conclusions. They call for greater clarity in reporting statistical process control charts along with greater adherence to methodological criteria. All this suggests a need for more training for those constructing charts and greater involvement of statistical process control experts.

4.2 Two Types of Errors When Using Statistical Process Control

Classifying variation into common cause or special cause is the primary focus of statistical process control methodology. In practice, this classification is subject to two types of error[4,13,15,28,45] (see Box 7) which can be compared to an imperfect screening test that sometimes shows a patient has disease when in fact the patient is free from disease (false positive), or the patient is free from disease when in fact the patient has disease (false negative).

Either error can cause losses. If all outcomes were treated as special cause variation, this maximises the losses from error 1. And if all outcomes were treated as common cause variation, this maximises the losses from error 2. Unfortunately, in practice, it is impossible to reduce both errors to zero and so a choice must be made to set the control limit. Shewhart concluded that it was best to make either error rarely and that this mainly depended upon how much it might cost to look for trouble in a stable process unnecessarily.[4,45] Using mathematical theory, empirical evidence, and pragmatism, he argued that setting control limits to ± three standard deviations from the mean provides a reasonable balance between making either type of error.

The choice of three standard deviations ensures there is a relatively small chance that an investigation of special cause variation will be unfounded because the chances of a false alarm are relatively low. The sensitivity (to special causes) could be increased by lowering the control limits to, say, two standard deviations. Although this will increase sensitivity, it will also increase the chances of false alarms. The extent to which this is acceptable requires decision-makers to balance the total costs (e.g. time, money, human resources, quality, safety, reputation) of investigating (true or false) signals versus the costs of overlooking these signals (and so not investigating). In practice, this is a matter of judgement which varies with context. Nevertheless, in the era of 'big data' in healthcare (see Section 4.6) the issue of false alarms needs greater appreciation and attention.

Box 7 Two types of error when using statistical process control

- Error 1: Treating an outcome resulting from a common cause as if it were a special cause and (wrongly) seeking to find a special cause, when in fact the cause is the underlying process.
- Error 2: Treating an outcome resulting from a special cause as if it were a common cause and so (wrongly) overlooking the special cause.

4.3 Using More Than One Statistical Process Control Chart

Although earlier sections have shown some examples of plotting more than one statistical process control chart for the same data, the literature tends to encourage people to identify the most appropriate single control chart. This offers a useful starting point, especially for beginners, but recognition is growing that use of two (or more) charts of the same data can offer useful insights that might not otherwise be noticed.[46,47]

For example, Figure 25 shows inspection data for the proportion of defective manufactured goods described by Deming.[45] The data are charted using two types of statistical process control chart: the p-chart (left panel) and the XmR chart (right panel). Each chart shows a central line and control limits at three standard deviations from the mean. While each chart appears to show common cause variation, marked differences in the width of the control limits across the two charts are evident. This suggests something unusual about these data. As Deming explains, these inspection figures were falsified (a special cause) because the inspector feared the plant would be closed if the proportion of defective goods went beyond 10%.[45] So, a systematic special cause has impacted all the data (not just a few data points), and that's why the limits between the two charts differ. This means that relying only on one chart risks overlooking the existence of this underlying special cause, whereas using two charts side by side provides additional insight.

Although decision-makers may not routinely have time and space to review multiple types of statistical control charts, analysts working with data might

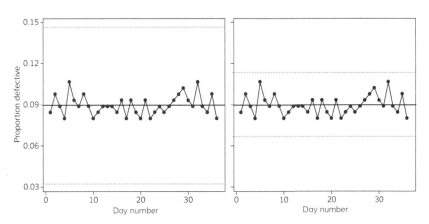

Figure 25 Two side-by-side statistical process control charts showing daily proportion of defective products. The left panel is a p-chart and the right panel is an XmR-chart. The difference in control limits indicates an underlying special cause even though each chart appears to be consistent with common cause variation when viewed alone

well seek to consider and explore the use of more than one chart. The additional insight gained could prove useful and requires little extra effort, especially if using software to produce the charts. Henderson et al.[47] suggest the combined use of run chart and CUSUM plots, and Rogers et al.[21] and Sherlaw-Johnson et al.[48] suggest the use of combined CUSUM-type charts.

4.4 The Risks of Risk-Adjusted Statistical Process Control in Healthcare

A distinctive feature of applying statistical process control in healthcare versus industry is the use of risk adjustment to reflect differences between patients.[13] Typically, this type of control chart relies on a statistical model to estimate the risk of death for a given patient and then compare this with the observed outcome (died or survived). When using risk-adjusted charts, the explanation for a signal of special cause variation might be thought to lie beyond the risk profile of the patient. But this approach is flawed: it fails to recognise that risk adjustment, although widely used in healthcare, is not a panacea and poses its own risks.[34,49–55]

For example, a systematic review of studies that examined the relationship between quality of care and risk-adjusted outcomes found counter-intuitive results: an 'intuitive' relationship (better care was associated with lower risk-adjusted death rates) was found in around half of the 52 relationships; the remainder showed either no correlation (there was no correlation between quality of care and risk-adjusted death rates) or a 'paradoxical' correlation (higher quality of care was associated with higher risk-adjusted death rates). The authors conclude that 'the link between quality of care and risk-adjusted mortality remains largely unreliable'. [51]

The consequences of prematurely inferring problems with the quality of care on the basis of casemix-adjusted statistical control charts can be serious (see Box 8).

Another crucial issue with risk-adjustment schemes is that they operate under the assumption of a constant relationship between patient risk factors and the outcome (e.g. between age and mortality). But if this relationship is not constant, then risk adjustment may increase rather than decrease[50,54] the very bias it was designed to overcome.

This misconception – that casemix-adjusted outcomes can be reliably used to blame quality of care – is termed the 'casemix adjustment fallacy'.[34] This bear trap can be avoided by adopting the Pyramid Model of investigation, described in Section 3.6, which underscores the point that casemix adjustment has its own risks, and that care needs to be taken when interpreting casemix-adjusted analyses.[34]

BOX 8 WRONGLY SUGGESTING THAT THE SPECIAL CAUSE VARIATION AFTER RISK
ADJUSTMENT IMPLIES PROBLEMS WITH QUALITY OF CARE

A renowned specialist hospital received a letter from the Care Quality
Commission informing them that a risk-adjusted hospital mortality
monitoring scheme had signalled an unacceptably high death rate: 27.8
deaths were expected, but 46 had been observed. In 2017, senior
hospital staff wrote in *The Lancet*:

> One might ask, however, what harm is done? After all, it is better to
> monitor than not and a hospital falsely accused of being a negative
> outlier can defend itself with robust data and performance monitoring.
> That is true but, because of this spurious alert, our hospital morale was
> shaken; management and trust board members were preoccupied with
> this issue for weeks; and our already stretched audit department
> expended over 50 person-hours of work reviewing data and formulat-
> ing a response to satisfy the Care Quality Commission that we are most
> certainly not a negative outlier, but a unit with cardiac results among
> the best in the country.[52]

Another example is the use of the Partial Risk Adjustment in Surgery
model, which fails to adjust for certain comorbid conditions and
underestimates the risk for the highest-risk patients. This reportedly led
to a negative impression of performance in one UK centre that was
involved in real-time monitoring of risk-adjusted paediatric cardiac
surgery outcomes (for procedures carried out during 2010 and 2011)
using variable life-adjusted display plots.[53]

4.5 Methodological Controversies in Statistical Process Control

Debates between methodologists on the correct way to think about the design
and use of statistical process control charts have been a long-standing feature of
the technical literature.[40] Our purpose here is not to review these issues, but
simply to highlight that these controversies have existed for decades. For
example, Nelson first wrote a note addressing five misconceptions relating to
Shewhart control charts (these are set out in Box 9) in 1999.[55]

In a similar vein, Blackstone's 2004 analysis provided a surgeon's critique of
the methodological issues of using risk-adjusted CUSUM charts to monitor
surgical performance.[56] One feature of CUSUM-based schemes is that they
appear to place considerably more emphasis on statistical significance testing
than Shewhart control charts. Blackstone notes that while most 'discussants'
agree that continual testing is 'in some sense' subject to the multiple

> Box 9 Five misconceptions that have led to methodological controversy in respect of Shewhart control charts[55]
>
> 1. Shewhart charts are a graphical way of applying a sequential statistical significance test for an out-of-control condition.
> 2. Control limits are confidence limits on the true process mean.
> 3. Shewhart charts are based on probabilistic models, subject to or involving chance variation.
> 4. Normality is required for the correct application of a mean (or x bar) chart.
> 5. The theoretical basis for the Shewhart control chart has some obscurities that are difficult to teach.
>
> Contrary to what is found in many articles and books, all five of these statements are incorrect.

comparisons problem, and one's interpretation must be affected by how often the data are evaluated, some statisticians maintain that the multiple comparison problem 'is not applicable to the quality control setting'. Blackstone goes on to say, 'I am not sure what to believe, frankly, nor do I think this issue will be soon resolved.' Happily, practitioners can profit from the use of statistical process control methodology without having to address these controversies.[40]

4.6 The Future of Statistical Process Control in Healthcare

The use of statistical process control to support efforts to monitor and improve the quality of healthcare is well established, with calls to extend its use.[57–60] Although it 'cannot solve all problems and must be applied wisely',[12] the future for statistical process control in healthcare looks promising, including wider use across clinical and managerial processes. However, the use of statistical process control methodology at scale presents some additional unique challenges.[61–63]

As an example, consider a hospital with five divisions, each with five wards: a single measure (such as staff absence) plotted on a control chart leads to 25 charts across the wards plus five charts across the divisions and one chart across the organisation (31 charts in total). Rolling out control charts across an entire organisation would require practical ways for staff to easily produce and collate charts (see Box 10).

Where there are thousands of control charts, users also need an effective way to collate them so they can still see the wood for the trees. This is an active area

Box 10 Scaling up control charts across East London NHS Foundation Trust[61]

East London NHS Foundation Trust (ELFT), established in 2000, provides mental health and community health services to a culturally diverse and socio-economically deprived catchment area of approximately 1.5 million people.

In 2014, ELFT launched its trust-wide quality improvement programme, which has adopted the Institute for Healthcare Improvement's Model for Improvement using tools such as PDSA cycles, driver diagrams, and statistical process control charts. This commitment developed from a desire to shift power in the organisation so that service users, carers, and staff were better able to understand and improve the quality of care being provided.

An important challenge was to capture the learning at team level. Teams recorded their PDSA tests of change locally using paper or local IT systems. This was not reliable, so, the IT team at ELFT developed an online quality improvement platform to make it much easier for teams to log their PDSAs, create driver diagrams, and input and view their data as control charts. The IT system supports the production of statistical process control charts which usually require fixing of baselines, recalculating limits following a successful change and annotations that highlight the changes. Given the scores of charts to choose from, the automation of charts overcomes an important barrier, especially for new users. The Inpatient Mental Health Analytics app has 34,650 statistical process control charts with over 100,000 charts across the organisation.

of research, involving proposals based on summary measures shown on a single graph to visualise the many control charts and spot the ones of most concern.[61–63]

A related issue is the massive proliferation of automatically collected digital data in healthcare.[64,65] It has been estimated that up to 30% of the entire world's stored data is health related.[65] This so-called big data is characterised by high volume (e.g. a single patient generates up to 80 megabytes of data annually, which is about 40,000 pages), high velocity (e.g. patient movement can be automatically collected every 30 seconds), and high variety (with multiple sources of data which include test results, images, text, movement, etc.). Although several researchers[66–68] have suggested that statistical process control charting may be useful to monitor big data over time, a number of methodological challenges need to be addressed, including the cautious choice of the sampling and collection interval.[69] For example, if data are available every second, then should these data be charted every second, minute, hour, and so on? Also, as more variables are monitored more often, it becomes increasingly important to keep the number of false alarms at a manageable number. A false alarm is a signal of special cause variation which is false; if there are too many false alarms, then the monitoring scheme becomes ineffective and discredited. The successful use of control charts in the era of big data will require low false-alarm rates.

So, while the future of statistical process control methodology appears promising, paradoxically, its use at scale needs to address some unique challenges.

5 Conclusions

Statistical process control methodology is based on a fundamental intuitive insight – that processes are subject to two sources of variation: common cause versus special cause. As the case studies show, this profound insight enables us to understand, monitor, and improve a wide range of processes, such as a person's handwritten signatures, a person's blood pressure, the results from surgery, the performance of hospitals, and the progress of a pandemic. The methodology offers a useful, robust, versatile, statistical, practical, and evidence-based approach, but its successful application requires overcoming technical and non-technical barriers. Numerous studies now demonstrate that such barriers are surmountable. This highlights the remarkable progress of statistical process control methodology from manufacturing industry in the 1920s to present-day healthcare.

6 Further Reading

Constructing Statistical Process Control Charts

- Mohammed et al.[17] – a step-by-step tutorial paper to show practitioners how to produce commonly used Shewhart control charts.
- Provost and Murray[15] – a comprehensive book that focuses on the use of statistical process control in healthcare with worked examples on how to produce a wide range of control charts.
- Rogers et al.[21] – an overview of the use of CUSUM-type plots that are commonly used to monitor outcomes in surgery.

Statistical Process Control Methodology in Healthcare

- Thor et al.[12] – a systematic review of the application of statistical process control in healthcare improvement that also highlights the barriers and enablers to successful use of these methods.

- Tennant et al.[7] – a systematic review of the use of control charts to monitor individual patients.

Methodological Challenges and Controversies

- Woodall[40] – discusses some of the key methodological controversies in statistical process control.
- Woodall and Faltin[68] – highlight some of the key challenges of using statistical process control at scale and how they might be overcome.

Contributors

Conflicts of interest

None.

Acknowledgements

I thank the peer reviewers for their insightful comments and recommendations to improve the Element. A list of peer reviewers is published at www.cam bridge.org/IQ-peer-reviewers. I would also like to thank Steve Flood and Claire Dipple for their help in preparing this Element.

Funding

This Element was funded by THIS Institute (The Healthcare Improvement Studies Institute, www.thisinstitute.cam.ac.uk). THIS Institute is strengthening the evidence base for improving the quality and safety of healthcare. THIS Institute is supported by a grant to the University of Cambridge from the Health Foundation – an independent charity committed to bringing about better health and healthcare for people in the United Kingdom.

About the Author

Mohammed Amin Mohammed is Emeritus Professor of Healthcare Quality and Effectiveness at the Faculty of Health Studies, University of Bradford, and Principal Consultant at the Strategy Unit. His main areas of interest are health-care quality, performance measurement and monitoring, and more generally health services research in primary and secondary care.

Creative Commons License

References

1. Cox JF, Schleier JG, Editors. *Theory of Constraints Handbook.* New York: McGraw-Hill; 2010.

2. Baxter, R, Lawton, R. The positive deviance approach. In: Dixon-Woods M, Brown K, Marjanovic S et al., editors. *Elements of Improving Quality and Safety in Healthcare.* Cambridge: Cambridge University Press; 2022. https://doi.org/10.1017/9781009237130.

3. Boaden R, Furnival J, Sharp C. The Institute for Healthcare Improvement approach. In: Dixon-Woods M, Brown K, Marjanovic S et al., editors. *Elements of Improving Quality and Safety in Healthcare.* Cambridge: Cambridge University Press; forthcoming.

4. Shewhart WA. *Economic Control of Quality of Manufactured Product.* New York: D Van Nostrand Company; 1931. (Reprinted by ASQC Quality Press, 1980).

5. American Society for Quality. Walter A. Shewhart: Father of statistical quality control. https://asq.org/about-asq/honorary-members/shewhart (accessed 28 June 2020).

6. Karkalousos P, Evangelopoulos A. The history of statistical quality control in clinical chemistry and haematology (1950–2010). *Int J Biomed Lab Sci* 2015; 4: 1–11.

7. Tennant R, Mohammed MA, Coleman JJ, Martin U. Monitoring patients using control charts: A systematic review. *Int J Qual Health Care* 2007; 19: 187–94. https://doi.org/10.1093/intqhc/mzm015.

8. Piccoli A, Rizzoni G, Tessarin C, et al. Long-term monitoring of renal transplant patients by a CUSUM test on serum creatinine. *Nephron* 1987; 47: 87–94. https://doi.org/10.1159/000184467.

9. Gibson PG, Wlodarczyk J, Hensley MJ, et al. Using quality-control analysis of peak expiratory flow recordings to guide therapy for asthma. *Ann Intern Med* 1995; 123: 488–92. https://doi.org/10.7326/0003-4819-123-7-199510010-00002.

10. Solodky C, Chen H, Jones PK, Katcher W, Neuhauser D. Patients as partners in clinical research: A proposal for applying quality improvement methods to patient care. *Med Care* 1998; 36(Suppl.): AS13–20. https://doi.org/10.1097/00005650-199808001-00003.

11. Suman G, Prajapati D. Control chart applications in healthcare: A literature review. *Int J Metrol Qual Eng* 2018; 9: 5. https://doi.org/10.1051/ijmqe/2018003.

12. Thor J, Lundberg J, Ask J, et al. Application of statistical process control in healthcare improvement: Systematic review. *BMJ Qual Saf* 2007; 16: 387–99. https://doi.org/10.3109/07434618.2011.653604.

13. Woodall WH, Adams BM, Benneyan JC. The use of control charts in healthcare. In: Faltin FW, Kenett RS, Ruggeri F, editors. *Statistical Methods in Healthcare*. Chichester: Wiley; 2012; 251–67.

14. Bolsin S, Colson M. The use of the Cusum technique in the assessment of trainee competence in new procedures. *Int J Qual Health Care* 2000; 12: 433–8. https://doi.org/10.1093/intqhc/12.5.433.

15. Provost LP, Murray SK. *The Health Care Data Guide: Learning from Data for Improvement*. San Francisco: Jossey-Bass; 2011.

16. Perla RJ, Provost LP, Murray SK. The run chart: A simple analytical tool for learning from variation in healthcare processes. *BMJ Qual Saf* 2011; 20: 46–51. http://dx.doi.org/10.1136/bmjqs.2009.037895.

17. Mohammed MA, Worthington P, Woodall WH. Plotting basic control charts: Tutorial notes for healthcare practitioners. *BMJ Qual Saf* 2008; 17:137–45. http://dx.doi.org/10.1136/qshc.2004.012047.

18. Noyez L. Control charts, Cusum techniques and funnel plots. A review of methods for monitoring performance in healthcare. *Interact Cardiovasc Thorac Surg* 2009; 9: 494–9. https://doi.org/10.1510/icvts.2009.204768.

19. Anhøj J, Olesen AV. Run charts revisited: A simulation study of run chart rules for detection of non-random variation in health care processes. *PLoS ONE* 2014; 9: e113825. https://doi.org/10.1371/journal.pone.0113825.

20. Anhøj J. Diagnostic value of run chart analysis: Using likelihood ratios to compare run chart rules on simulated data series. *PLoS ONE* 2015; 10: e0121349. https://doi.org/10.1371/journal.pone.0121349.

21. Rogers CA, Reeves BC, Caputo M, et al. Control chart methods for monitoring cardiac surgical performance and their interpretation. *J Thorac Cardiovasc Surg* 2004; 128: 811–9. https://doi.org/10.1016/j.jtcvs.2004.03.011.

22. Silvester KM, Mohammed MA, Harriman P, Girolami A, Downes TW. Timely care for frail older people referred to hospital improves efficiency and reduces mortality without the need for extra resources. *Age Ageing* 2014; 43: 472–7. https://doi.org/10.1093/ageing/aft170.

23. Hebert C, Neuhauser D. Improving hypertension care with patient-generated run charts: Physician, patient, and management perspectives. *Qual Manag Health Care* 2004; 13: 174–7. https://doi.org/10.1097/00019514-200407000-00004.

24. Macpherson GJ, Brenkel IJ, Smith R, Howie CR. Outlier analysis in orthopaedics: Use of CUSUM. The Scottish arthroplasty project:

Shouldering the burden of improvement. *J Bone Joint Surg* 2011; 93(Suppl. 3): 81–8. https://doi.org/10.2106/JBJS.K.01010.

25. Duclos A, Chollet F, Pascal L, et al. Effect of monitoring surgical outcomes using control charts to reduce major adverse events in patients: Cluster randomised trial. *BMJ* 2020; 371: m3840. https://doi.org/10.1136/bmj.m3840.

26. Duclos A, Voirin N. The *p*-control chart: A tool for care improvement. *Int J Qual Health Care* 2010; 22: 402–7. https://doi.org/10.1093/intqhc/mzq037.

27. Spiegelhalter DJ. Funnel plots for comparing institutional performance. *Stat Med* 2005; 24: 1185–202. https://doi.org/10.1002/sim.1970.

28. Mohammed MA, Cheng KK, Rouse A, Marshall T. Bristol, Shipman, and clinical governance: Shewhart's forgotten lessons. *Lancet* 2001; 357: 463–7. https://doi.org/10.1016/S0140-6736(00)04019-8.

29. Verburg IW, Holman R, Peek N, Abu-Hanna A, de Keizer NF. Guidelines on constructing funnel plots for quality indicators: A case study on mortality in intensive care unit patients. *Stat Methods Med Res* 2018; 27: 3350–66. https://doi.org/10.1177%2F0962280217700169.

30. Guthrie B, Love T, Fahey T, Morris A, Sullivan F. Control, compare and communicate: Designing control charts to summarise efficiently data from multiple quality indicators. *BMJ Qual Saf* 2005; 14: 450–4. https://doi.org/10.1136/qshc.2005.014456.

31. Mayer EK, Bottle A, Rao C, Darzi AW, Athanasiou T. Funnel plots and their emerging application in surgery. *Ann Surg* 2009; 249(3): 376–83. https://doi.org/10.1097/SLA.0b013e31819a47b1.

32. Riley S, Burhouse A, Nicholas T. National Health Service (NHS) trust boards adopt statistical process control reporting: The impact of the making data count training programme. *BMJ Lead* 2021; 5: 252–7. http://dx.doi.org/10.1136/leader-2020-000357.

33. Kennedy I. *The Report of the Public Inquiry into Children's Heart Surgery at the Bristol Royal Infirmary 1984–1995. Learning from Bristol.* London: HMSO; 2001. www.bristol-inquiry.org.uk/final_report/index.htm (accessed September 2023).

34. Lilford R, Mohammed MA, Spiegelhalter D, Thomson R. Use and misuse of process and outcome data in managing performance of acute medical care: Avoiding institutional stigma. *Lancet* 2004; 363: 1147–54. https://doi.org/10.1016/S0140-6736(04)15901-1.

35. Mohammed MA, Rathbone A, Myers P, et al. An investigation into general practitioners associated with high patient mortality flagged up through the

Shipman inquiry: Retrospective analysis of routine data. *BMJ* 2004; 328: 1474 https://doi.org/10.1136/bmj.328.7454.1474.

36. Smith IR, Garlick B, Gardner MA et al. Use of graphical statistical process control tools to monitor and improve outcomes in cardiac surgery. *Heart Lung Circ* 2013; 22: 92–9. https://doi.org/10.1016/j.hlc.2012.08.060.

37. Mohammed MA, Booth K, Marshall D, et al. A practical method for monitoring general practice mortality in the UK: Findings from a pilot study in a health board of Northern Ireland. *Br J Gen Pract* 2005; 55: 670–6.

38. Duckett SJ, Coory M, Sketcher-Baker K. Identifying variations in quality of care in Queensland hospitals. *Med J Aust* 2007; 187: 571–5. https://doi.org/10.5694/j.1326-5377.2007.tb01419.x.

39. Schmidtke KA, Poots AJ, Carpio J, et al. Considering chance in quality and safety performance measures: An analysis of performance reports by boards in English NHS trusts. *BMJ Qual Saf* 2017; 26: 61–9. http://dx.doi.org/10.1136/bmjqs-2015-004967.

40. Woodall WH. Controversies and contradictions in statistical process control. *J Qual Technol* 2000; 32: 341–50. https://doi.org/10.1080/00224065.2000.11980013.

41. East London NHS Foundation Trust. Board of Directors Meeting in Public. Thursday 30 March 2023. www.elft.nhs.uk/sites/default/files/2023-03/Combined%20Public%20Trust%20Board%20-%20March%202023%20%28v001%29.pdf (accessed May 2023).

42. Perla RJ, Provost SM, Parry GJ, Little K, Provost LP. Understanding variation in covid-19 reported deaths with a novel Shewhart chart application. *Int J Qual Health Care* 2020; 33(1). https://doi.org/10.1093/intqhc/mzaa069.

43. Parry G, Provost LP, Provost SM, Little K, Perla RJ. A hybrid Shewhart chart for visualising and learning from epidemic data. *Int J Qual Health Care* 2021; 33: 1–10. https://doi.org/10.1093/intqhc/mzab151.

44. Koetsier A, van der Veer SN, Jager KJ, Peek N, de Keizer NF. Control charts in healthcare quality improvement: A systematic review on adherence to methodological criteria. *Methods Inf Med* 2012; 51: 189–98. https://doi.org/10.3414/ME11-01-0055.

45. Deming WE. *Out of the Crisis*. Cambridge, MA: MIT Press; 1986.

46. Mohammed MA, Worthington P. Why traditional statistical process control charts for attribute data should be viewed alongside an *xmr*-chart. *BMJ Qual Saf* 2013; 22: 263–9. http://dx.doi.org/10.1136/bmjqs-2012-001324.

47. Henderson GR, Davies R, Macdonald D. Bringing data to life with post-hoc CUSUM charts. *Case Studies Bus Ind Gov Stats* 2010; 3: 60–9.

48. Sherlaw-Johnson C, Morton A, Robinson MB, Hall A. Real-time monitoring of coronary care mortality: A comparison and combination of two monitoring tools. *Int J Cardiol* 2005; 100: 301–7. https://doi.org/10.1016/j.ijcard.2004.12.009.

49. Iezzoni LI. The risks of risk adjustment. *JAMA* 1997; 278: 1600–7. https://doi.org/10.1001/jama.1997.03550190064046.

50. Nicholl J. Case-mix adjustment in non-randomised observational evaluations: The constant risk fallacy. *J Epidemiol Community Health* 2007; 61: 1010–3. http://dx.doi.org/10.1136/jech.2007.061747.

51. Pitches DW, Mohammed MA, Lilford RJ. What is the empirical evidence that hospitals with higher-risk adjusted mortality rates provide poorer quality care? A systematic review of the literature. *BMC Health Serv Res* 2007; 7: 91. https://doi.org/10.1186/1472-6963-7-91.

52. Nashef SA, Powell S, Jenkins DP, Fynn S, Hall R. Crying wolf: The misuse of hospital data. *Lancet* 2017; 390: 227–8. https://doi.org/10.1016/S0140-6736(17)31609-4.

53. O'Neill S, Wigmore SJ, Harrison EM. Debate: Should we use variable adjusted life displays (VLAD) to identify variations in performance in general surgery? *BMC Surg* 2015; 15: 102. https://doi.org/10.1186/s12893-015-0087-0.

54. Mohammed MA, Deeks JJ, Girling A, et al. Evidence of methodological bias in hospital standardised mortality ratios: Retrospective database study of English hospitals. *BMJ* 2009; 338: b780. https://doi.org/10.1136/bmj.b780.

55. Nelson LS. Notes on the Shewhart control chart. *J Qual Tech* 1999; 31: 124–6. https://doi.org/10.1080/00224065.1999.11979903.

56. Blackstone EH. Monitoring surgical performance. *J Thorac Cardiovasc Surg* 2004; 128: 807–10. https://doi.org/10.1016/j.jtcvs.2004.03.022.

57. O'Brien T, Viney R, Doherty A, Thomas K. Why don't Mercedes Benz publish randomized trials? *BJUI* 2010; 105: 293–5. https://doi.org/10.1111/j.1464-410X.2009.09000.x.

58. Polit DF, Chaboyer W. Statistical process control in nursing research. *Res Nurs Health* 2012; 35: 82–93. https://doi.org/10.1002/nur.20467.

59. Fretheim A, Tomic O. Statistical process control and interrupted time series: A golden opportunity for impact evaluation in quality improvement. *BMJ Qual Saf* 2015; 24: 748–52. http://dx.doi.org/10.1136/bmjqs-2014-003756.

60. O'Sullivan OP, Chang NH, Baker P, Shah A. Quality improvement at East London NHS foundation trust: The pathway to embedding lasting change. *Int J Health Govern* 2021; 26: 65–72. https://doi.org/10.1108/IJHG-07-2020-0085.

61. Jensen WA, Szarka III J, White K. Stability assessment with the stability index. *Qual Eng* 2019; 31: 289–301. https://doi.org/10.1080/08982112 .2018.1497179.

62. Sall J. Scaling-up process characterization. *Qual Eng* 2018; 30: 62–78. https://doi.org/10.1080/08982112.2017.1361539.

63. Suter-Crazzolara C. Better patient outcomes through mining of biomedical big data. *Front ICT* 2018; 5: 30. https://doi.org/10.3389/fict.2018.00030.

64. Gopal G, Suter-Crazzolara C, Toldo L, Eberhardt W. Digital transformation in healthcare–architectures of present and future information technologies. *Clin Chem Lab Med* 2019; 57: 328–35. https://doi.org/10.1515/cclm-2018-0658.

65. Qiu P. Big data? Statistical process control can help! *Amer Statistician* 2020; 74: 329–44. https://doi.org/10.1080/00031305.2019.1700163.

66. Megahed FM, Jones-Farmer LA. Statistical perspectives on 'big data'. In: Knoth S, Schmid W, editors. *Frontiers in Statistical Quality Control 11*. Cham: Springer; 2015: 29–47. https://doi.org/10.1007/978-3-319-12355-4_3.

67. Qiu P. Statistical process control charts as a tool for analyzing big data. In: Ahmed SE, editor. *Big and Complex Data Analysis: Methodologies and Applications*. Cham: Springer; 2017: 123–38. https://doi.org/10.1007/978-3-319-41573-4_7.

68. Woodall WH, Faltin FW. Rethinking control chart design and evaluation. *Qual Eng* 2019; 31: 596–605. https://doi.org/10.1080/08982112.2019 .1582779.

69. Zwetsloot IM, Woodall WH. A review of some sampling and aggregation strategies for basic statistical process monitoring. *J Qual Technol* 2021; 53: 1–16. https://doi.org/10.1080/00224065.2019.1611354.

Cambridge Elements ☰

Improving Quality and Safety in Healthcare

Editors-in-Chief

Mary Dixon-Woods

THIS Institute (The Healthcare Improvement Studies Institute)

Mary is Director of THIS Institute and is the Health Foundation Professor of Healthcare Improvement Studies in the Department of Public Health and Primary Care at the University of Cambridge. Mary leads a programme of research focused on healthcare improvement, healthcare ethics, and methodological innovation in studying healthcare.

Graham Martin

THIS Institute (The Healthcare Improvement Studies Institute)

Graham is Director of Research at THIS Institute, leading applied research programmes and contributing to the institute's strategy and development. His research interests are in the organisation and delivery of healthcare, and particularly the role of professionals, managers, and patients and the public in efforts at organisational change.

Executive Editor

Katrina Brown

THIS Institute (The Healthcare Improvement Studies Institute)

Katrina was Communications Manager at THIS Institute, providing editorial expertise to maximise the impact of THIS Institute's research findings. She managed the project to produce the series until 2023.

Editorial Team

Sonja Marjanovic

RAND Europe

Sonja is Director of RAND Europe's healthcare innovation, industry, and policy research. Her work provides decision-makers with evidence and insights to support innovation and improvement in healthcare systems, and to support the translation of innovation into societal benefits for healthcare services and population health.

Tom Ling

RAND Europe

Tom is Head of Evaluation at RAND Europe and President of the European Evaluation Society, leading evaluations and applied research focused on the key challenges facing health services. His current health portfolio includes evaluations of the innovation landscape, quality improvement, communities of practice, patient flow, and service transformation.

Ellen Perry

THIS Institute (The Healthcare Improvement Studies Institute)

Ellen supported the production of the series during 2020–21.

Gemma Petley

THIS Institute (The Healthcare Improvement Studies Institute)
Gemma is Senior Communications and Editorial Manager at THIS Institute, responsible for overseeing the production and maximising the impact of the series.

Claire Dipple

THIS Institute (The Healthcare Improvement Studies Institute)
Claire is Editorial Project Manager at THIS Institute, responsible for editing and project managing the series.

About the Series

The past decade has seen enormous growth in both activity and research on improvement in healthcare. This series offers a comprehensive and authoritative set of overviews of the different improvement approaches available, exploring the thinking behind them, examining evidence for each approach, and identifying areas of debate.

Cambridge Elements $\overline{\overline{}}$

Improving Quality and Safety in Healthcare